Sleep

Effective and Proven Tips to Improving Your Sleeping Routine

By
Faye Froome

Faye Froome Copyright © 2016

Table of Contents

Introduction

Thanks for buying this book, we hope it goes someway to helping you get the sleep you need and deserve after a busy day.

Sleep is important, we don't get enough of it and we should seek to get more, and of a better quality. How you feel during the waking hours hinges greatly on how you slept the evening before.

Sleep is one of the most overlooked things we can do for ourselves in order to better our health. As we digest more and more media we are constantly bombarded with health warnings linked to diet, alcohol, smoking, and lack of exercise. All of these things are of course important to our health and should be taken notice of. It's not surprising that many of us when we think of getting healthy we focus first and foremost on diet and exercise. Diet and exercise are important to us but if we focused more upon our quality of sleep then we can make diet and exercise work better for us.

At first sight, it might seem that sleep is a completely natural phenomenon, a way in which our bodies regulate their own health and rhythm. This is fundamentally true, because sleep is a state the human body needs in order to function properly. However, many people ignore the fact that they can actually improve the quality of their sleep. What does this mean exactly? Does good sleep only come down to a number of hours? Do you think the more you sleep, the better you feel?

Although sleeping for an optimal number of hours is definitely important, we must not ignore other factors that contribute to the quality of our sleep such as diet, lifestyle, or the sleeping environment.

This book is a short guide to understanding the numerous benefits of sleep for your health and to discovering the best methods of enhancing your sleep and thus leading a more healthy life. In this book, you will find out why it's vital to get a good sleep and what you can do to ensure you sleep better. A good night sleep doesn't only result in high energy and effective performance on the following day. Many of us might think sleep will only affect their capacity or their tiredness after they wake up. In fact, many of us ignore the long-term benefits of sleep for our health as well as the more subtle ways a good night's sleep can improve various systems in our bodies. It's not only a matter of feeling relaxed or feeling tired during the following day. The effects of our sleep (and of its high or lacking quality) are pervasive and somewhat insidious. How exactly your sleep can affect your health is something you will discover in the following chapter. So read on and learn to master your own sleep in order to lead a better life!

The Health Benefits of Sleep You May Not Know about

Ok so we all know what sleep is, but do we really know what happens to us while we are in the land of nod? Far from being just a state of unconsciousness our bodies go through a whole raft of processes that enable us to function effectively as a human being through our waking hours.

Sleeping is a period of rest that enables the body to detoxify and undergo essential repair. Poor sleeping patterns equate to poor health for many of us. It has been suggested by health experts that people who sleep for 5 hours or less have a shorter life expectancy than those that get over 6 hours sleep a night. So as we can see sleep has a very important role to play in our physical and mental wellbeing.

Although we are lying still (mostly) and in a dormant state the brain remains very active during our time asleep, of course not as active as we when we are awake, but nonetheless our brain activity is still around the 60% of our normal activity.

Research has shown that our brain enters various cycles with varying degrees of brain waves that transmit signals to different parts of our bodies during our sleep. The two main stages are Non rapid eye movement (NREM) and rapid eye movement (REM). In all there are 5 stages of sleep that occur throughout NREM and REM.

During NREM which accounts for about 75% of our night sleep we encounter 4 stages of sleep. The first stage is basically nodding off, this includes us going to bed and relaxing through to a light sleep when we first fall asleep.

The second stage is us falling to sleep properly, our heart rate becomes regular and our body temperature drops. We also become less aware of our surroundings as we enter a state of unconsciousness.

This leads us into stage 3 and 4 of our sleep pattern. Here we find ourselves in the deepest sleep of the evening. Our blood pressure drops and our breathing slows right down. This is the most crucial part of our sleep as so much of the restorative work is done by the brain and body. Our muscles become relaxed leading to increased blood flow into these areas resulting in tissues damage to be repaired. At this point our energy levels are also being restored to enable to face the coming waking hours. Hormones at this stage are also released, if we are in our formative younger years, these hormones encourage growth of our body.

The next and final stage is what is known as REM. Even though our eyes are closed underneath the eyes are making darting rapid movements. Out brain activity is at its highest point during this stage and it's when we are most likely to dream. We also have bouts of irregular breathing and our heart rate becomes irregular too. However during this period our muscles are paralyzed preventing voluntary muscle movement.

The above 5 phases can also be broken down into another 3 phases of sleep that are outlined below.

Energy Conservation, Restoration, and Brain Plasticity

First and foremost, sleep helps your body recharge by means of a complex process of energy conservation. Harvard University researchers have highlighted three main functions of sleep: energy conservation, body rejuvenation, and brain plasticity. These notions may sound quite abstract and hard to grasp at a glance, but you have surely noticed their effects on your health yourself. During sleep, your energy demand and expenditure are reduced. This process is natural both in humans and animals. When we sleep, our metabolism is reduced and as such our body can conserve energy resources.

Although it might seem to be one and the same process, restoration is another effect of sleep. Our body spends energy and gets 'used up' through the normal activities we engage in while we are awake. We're talking both energy and cell structure here. If you want to have a clear picture of the rejuvenating function of sleep, just think about your muscle force when you are extremely tired and compare it with your tonus after a good sleep. Similarly, you can notice the revitalizing effects of sleep on your skin. Cell rejuvenation is actually one of the most significant effects of a good sleep and this takes place on many levels of your body and mind.

It's not only the beauty of your skin that can be improved by means of quality sleep, but also your immunity. Did you know that animals are prone to dying if deprived of sleep for a long time? This explains through the relation between sleep and the immune function. At the same time, your hormonal balance is regulated during your sleep. Your sleep provides the terrain for many essential processes in your body. For instance, protein synthesis occurs during our sleep.

Another significant effect of sleep that Harvard scientists examined is brain plasticity. This phenomenon is more sophisticated and it has to do with the discovery that sleep improves the structure and organization of our brain processes in very subtle ways. The main factor that contributes to this is stage known as REM. Our dreams allow our brains to engage in elaborate processes that mimic real-life scenarios and activities. Thus REM allows for a high degree of creativity and plasticity. Our capacity to dream and the things that happen in our consciousness as we sleep enhance our brain's general plasticity and potential to perform various types of tasks during the day. Keep in mind that our brain doesn't simply sink into a state of complete inaction during sleep! It continues to act 'on its own' and stream various films in our heads. This state of unconscious, but quite complex activity that also follows some logic of its own is known to improve our brain's capacity of focusing on many different types of tasks during the day. It's as if your brain practiced silently as you sleep!

Hormonal Activity

Apart from these rather general health benefits of sleep, there are many ways in which the quality and duration of your sleep can help you live better and longer. A highly important factor is the release and enhancement of various hormones in the body during sleep. For instance, the widely known and essential growth hormone is meant to help our body develop during sleep. That's why children sleep a lot – their growth is directly linked to this process in the body.

However, the growth hormone also helps adults. The better you sleep, the more you can avoid muscle atrophy and the more alive you keep your cells and tissues. This aspect might not be visible right away, of course. It's hard to tell if your muscles are strong or weak only after 8 hours of sleep. However, you should keep in mind the long-term effects of a good sleep. If you succeed in improving your sleep regularly and you benefit from all its advantages, the condition of your tissues will certainly be better.

This is a scientifically proven fact attributed to the release of various hormones during sleep time. Similarly, even sex hormones increase during sleep, which will lead to a boost in sexual energy and desire. For men this aspect can have quite an important effect when it comes to sexual dysfunctions. Some people might have already noticed that lack of sleep can cause erectile dysfunction and lower the libido. A great sleep will also regulate your sex hormones and implicitly your overall sex life.

Memory and Learning

One of the most interesting and far-reaching benefits of excellent sleep involves our memory and learning capacity. Of course, we all know that we have done better in exams or presentations after many hours of sound sleep. However, a good sleeping routine will improve your general memory and learning potential. The effects might be less obvious right away, but powerful nonetheless. Research indicates that sleep interferes with our memory processes and the way we perceive or recall events or data.

This is important from several points of view: sleep can help you 'store' facts that you should remember, but also organize information better so that you can access and use it when needed. At the same time, good sleep helps your memory in a more emotional sense: your general mood, state of mind, and even perception and understanding of events can be affected by the kind of sleep you have.

When you are tired, your mind might run adrift and make you recall mainly negative events, which put you in a bad mood. That's why a good sleep is recommendable for the ability to judge things objectively and ensure your memory is free of excessive emotional bias. Sleep plays a major part in the storing/consolidation stage of our memory processes. You acquire facts and you pull them out of your memory for concrete usage as you are awake. However, data storage and organization have proven to be enhanced by high quality sleep – that's what scientists tell us. As for learning and performance, both immediate factors and long-term routine are at play here: when you get a good sleep, you can perform better in school or at work.

Your attention, your concentration power, your vigilance, and your ability to operate with data are much better after excellent sleep. However getting good sleep on a regular basis will also influence our mental capacities and our ability to perform task and learn new information. Our brain simply becomes more 'relaxed' and permissive to new facts which we can store unconsciously in a better structured way. All we have to do is make sure we know what good sleep means and we can improve our memory and learning abilities!

Sharp Focus and Fast Decision-making

Better sleep will help you in any situation that requires sharp focus and fast decision-making e.g. driving, sports, contests, exams etc. Scientists claim lack of sleep can even impact our brain in a way similar to alcohol ingestion. Thus any context that requires vigilance and mental swiftness is likely to be positively influenced by quality sleep – from business deals to contests or job interviews. Last, but not least, a higher mental capacity is accompanied by a better verbal performance when you get soothing sleep. People who sleep well are more articulate and fluent. So consider this important aspect of your 'night life' when you see you could do better in presentations or performances.

Skin Health

One of the most precious benefits of sleep is skin health. Sleep rejuvenates your tissues and can help you alleviate wrinkles and dark circles. Sleep can be soothing for dry skin and it can also help your skin cure from within – basically many unwanted skin conditions from irritation or sunburn to pimples can decrease if you get a sound and long sleep. Your skin learns to 'recycle' its own cells during sleep. Of course, you should also apply regular forms of skin care. Just don't forget how important sleep is!

Stress Relief and Emotional Regulator

People who sleep well can cope with stress much better. They judge things more clearly and are able to stay calm even in tense situations. Better sleep helps you avoid emotions such as anxiety, anger, or indignation, which will definitely improve your relationships and your performance at work. Simultaneously a sound sleep balances your mood and helps you get rid of depressive states of mind or panic attacks. In other words, sleep is like an emotional regulator that works independently of your conscious processes. Of course, if you are going through a hard time, you are encouraged to seek professional help or resort to additional solutions for your condition. However, keep in mind that better sleep could also help you get rid of negative emotions or irritability.

Soothing Various Types of Illness

Sleep doesn't only free you from stress, but it can also soothe migraines by allowing your body and brain to heal. It's a proven fact that people who don't get enough sleep report more headaches than the rest. Although this should be taken with a grain of salt, some studies also suggest good sleep can help you in dealing with more serious health problems such as diabetes or heart problems. Apparently a sound slumber can decrease blood pressure, which also lowers the risk of heart attack. For this reason, people who suffer from heart problems should make sure they sleep well and long enough. Around 8-9 hours of sleep per night are the guarantee of a healthy heart. Sleep is also said to regulate cholesterol, not only heart pressure, which is a sure way to counter or avoid heart disease.

A Tool in Cancer Prevention

An effect of excellent sleep may be even keeping the risk of cancer at bay, as unbelievable as it may sound on a first impression. When cancer is such a harsh enemy, how could it be kept away with so easy and accessible a weapon? Well, certainly if someone is already ill, sleep alone will not help too much. However, a long-term routine of perfect sleep is said to help people in this respect. During sleep (especially if you sleep in complete darkness) the levels of melatonin in your body increase, which inhibits the growth of tumorous cells on the long run. Thus a great habit of healthy sleep can indeed help you avoid cancer, especially colon and breast cancer.

Hormone Activation

As you have already noticed, many hormones find a propitious terrain in your sleep. It sounds quite easy, doesn't it? Hormones in your body are activated more while you do nothing at all. That's why you can also lose weight or at least stay fit by sleeping. In case you wonder if it's a joke – the answer is no. Studies have shown that people who sleep well and long enough are more likely to stay thin, because sleep increases the production of leptin in your body.

Do you how many people (especially women) struggle to get this hormone to higher levels and lose weight? Leptin is responsible for appetite regulation and it's usually associated with an effective kind of weight loss that can have long-term reliability. So getting your sleep routines to a level of excellence is quite important if you want to stay fit without much effort! Studies say people who don't get over 7-8 hours of sleep per night might have lower levels of leptin and thus suffer from unwanted weight problems.

Another hormone that is released during our sleep is cortisol. When cortisol levels are low, your skin is more exposed to wrinkles, fine lines, and lack of tonus. Cortisol helps your body break down the collagen proteins that are involved in the aging processes of your skin. Together with the growth hormone, cortisol and collagen are quite important to skin health. Thus sleeping well and more can help you keep your skin young through a stimulation of the right hormones in your body.

As you can see, there are myriad reasons why you should do your best to get better sleep. Not only can your overall health improve through an enhancement of your immunity processes and body revitalization, but also you can easily secure a positive emotional state by means of good sleep.

In more simple terms, better sleep can actually help you to grow happier and more invulnerable to stress or disease by encouraging several natural processes through which your body protects, maintains, or repairs itself. From stronger focus and memory to a younger and healthier body, all the benefits this chapter showed you are definitely worth the effort of changing your sleep routines for your own good.

How should you do this? Is it complicated? Are other areas of your life involved as well? You will find answers to such questions in the next chapter which will advise you about the optimal methods for sleep improvement and give you a series of tips and tricks you can use if you want to get better sleep.

Top Tips to Better Sleep

What does it take to get into a habit of good sleep through your own actions and measures? Can we control or manage our sleep? Or is everything up to more subtle organic processes in our body and we can just enjoy our sleep … or bear the consequences of insomnia? This chapter will help you push through your sleep problems by providing you with many tips to improving your sleep routine.

People who have chronic sleep disorders are advised to seek professional help before practicing the techniques this book introduces. Such tips are definitely beneficial for everyone. However, more severe disorders that affect one's life drastically should be addressed first and foremost through the advice of a medical specialist.

Additionally such people can always resort to the methods introduced in this book in order to increase their chances of success. The tips you will find in this chapter are meant primarily for people who suffer from mild to moderate or apparently random sleep problems. If you want to sleep more hours per night, if you have trouble falling asleep, or if you feel you don't always wake up relaxed and energetic, this book will provide you with all the help you need!

So how can you take control of your sleep? The most important thing to keep in mind before you go through the tips in this book is the fact that it's far more recommendable to try to incorporate several techniques into your life. Just respecting one "rule", but ignoring many other aspects involved in a healthy sleep will guarantee you much less than going for a holistic approach.

What does this mean? Essentially, you will have more chances of actual success if you consider your diet, your sleeping environment, your energy management, your daily routines, your mood, your hygiene etc. You should try to reach a broad picture that takes into account many factors that can affect your sleep. Addressing many aspects of your life is the path to better sleep and more health.

Sleep Duration

For starters, keep in mind that the best duration of your sleep is 8-9 hours. This is the time frame you should aim at. If you happen to feel tired and lethargic, start by asking yourself how many hours you allow yourself to sleep. Keep track of your daily schedule and avoid sleeping only when you have enough time at hands.

All of us had periods of high stress and heavy workload that might have forced us to decrease the duration of our sleep for a few days. Nevertheless, this is not a habit to follow. Such a thing shouldn't happen regularly out of ignorance, negligence, or bravado. Sleep should be like a ritual of your body, one that you don't only practice because you have to. Sleep is not something to squeeze in your schedule. Treat your sleep routines wisely and carefully.

Diet Tips

Is there anything you can include in your diet to facilitate your sleep? Although food is only a small part of a good sleep program, you should know there are certain plants that can help you sleep better. Valerian, melissa, passion fruit, chamomile, lavender, and elder are just a few of the most well-known plants that you can use for a sound sleep.

The easiest way is to prepare tea and drink it a little time before going to bed. Keep in mind however that you might want to avoid filling your stomach with tea if you want to sleep undisturbed. Ideally, you should drink your tea 1-2 hours before going to bed. Alternatively, you can purchase the plants in the form of powder or capsules, since they are very concentrated and easier to digest without too much liquid.

As for food that can help you sleep, the most famous is onion. "Unbelievable!", you might think. How could such bland and 'raw' food be an actual cure for insomnia? Well, while it is not actually the strongest remedy for sleep disorders, onion is surely a rather "traditionally valued" trick that can cause sleepiness and ease your way through slumber. Usually a rather problematic ingredient due to its taste and smell, onion is easy to use and digest at night when you only have to sleep, isn't it? It's enough if you combine it with your usual food for dinner (especially if you eat later in the evening). You should however eat at least 1/2-2/3 of an onion in order to make sure it has an effect on your body and mind.

There is also food you can consume on a regular basis in order to improve your sleep. Their effect won't be as immediate as in the previous case, but the content and the nutrients it brings in your body will prove to be effective on a longer run through a rather slow and sure action.

What can you include in your diet if you want to sleep better? Walnuts are well-known for their high amount of tryptophan, an amino acid that is important in the production of melatonin, the hormone that regulates your sleep. Almonds and bananas as a great source of magnesium, which is an amazing resource when it comes to stress relief and regulating the body's need and capacity for rest and relaxation. Garlic, tuna, and pistachio nuts are your sure weapons in combating insomnia, because they contain high amounts of vitamin B6 which has proven very useful in the production of melatonin, your "sleep hormone".

Another food that boosts melatonin is cherry. You can eat raw cherries or natural cherry juice – both will have the desired effect. Kale is a plant that is very rich in calcium, which allows tryptophan to synthesize melatonin easier. Hummus, cereals, rice, and whole grains can have the same effect of increasing the levels of tryptophan in your body.

In case you wonder why you cannot simply take in melatonin pills in order to regulate your sleep life more easily, the answer is actually not complicated: artificial hormone intake is likely to give you an apparent 'boost' for a short while after which you are prone to returning to your sleep problems.

If medical investigations prove that you have a serious melatonin deficit, then you should follow medical advice and regulate your hormone levels by other means. However, if you only feel tired and you cannot always sleep as you should, it's wiser to try to balance your body through a milder and more reliable method such as diet. Introducing the right food and nutrients in your diet will certainly have long-term benefits and no side effects.

People usually take melatonin when they change their time zone and they must learn to sleep at different hours or when they really suffer from diagnosed problems in the production and synthesis of this hormone. Otherwise it's perfect if you just stimulate the production of melatonin and add other minerals, vitamins, and nutrients in your body that are likely to help you sleep better.

How about what you shouldn't drink or eat? First of all, we all know that coffee is quite good for energy throughout the day, but ideally you should avoid it after 4pm if you want to have an undisturbed sleep by 11-12pm. Some people may think you shouldn't drink coffee in the evening if you want to sleep.

However, things are not so easy, as caffeine will gather in your body for hours and affect your sleep. You should also avoid coke, green tea, black tea, and various stimulants/energizing drinks if you want to sleep well. Ideally, you should drink them only in the morning and around noon. How about alcohol? While you might think a beer or a glass of wine might level your path to sleep, you should be very careful with a larger quantity. Alcohol actually unbalances processes in your body and can inhibit your sleep considerably if you yield to excesses. Similarly, you should stay away from nicotine or other addictions you might have. Some things might only leave the impression they help you relax, but actually affect your sleep on a deeper level.

When it comes to both food and drink, you should avoid stuffing your stomach with too much when you want to go to bed. Avoid having dinner too late (after 7pm) if you go to bed early. Allow your food to digest easily before you start your night routine. Don't drink too much liquid (of any kind) before you go to bed. You digestive system should be light and relaxed, too, if you want your nervous system to work properly towards a good sleep. Remember that systems and processes in your body don't act independently, but they are rather connected in more or less subtle ways.

Activities and Lifestyle that Encourage Good Sleep

What should you do before going to bed in order to ensure a soft and sound sleep? Ideally, you should avoid demanding and excessively energizing activities such as hard work, problem-solving, workouts, complicated or disturbing movies, "hard and heavy" music etc. Apart from activities that might usually fit your needs or mood, but are prone to interfering with the mental energy you need for rest, you should stay away from highly charged conversations or emotional exchanges. For instance, avoid fighting over negative things or debating problematic issues before going to be.

If there are people whose energy you perceive as negative and harsh, you can avoid interacting with them when you want to rest. Only engage in peaceful and fulfilling activities. The best way to ease your sleep is to listen to chill and pleasant music, read a few pages from a light book in bed, watch a romantic comedy or a documentary about places and phenomena that are accessible and positive etc.

How about television? Although some programs can be quite relaxing, for technical reasons it's better to avoid watching it before going to bed. You can watch a film on your tablet with a much softer light or you can resort to audio books.

Writing down a few things in a diary could also work for better sleep, as it helps you release energy accumulated during the day. Use a classic notebook and pen while you are already in bed and simply let your thoughts flow on the paper. Don't try to be too elaborate or sophisticated.

It's the act in itself that matters here – not the "literary' result. That's why it's irrelevant if you fall asleep as you write a sentence. Letting your stream of consciousness enter a rather natural flow will evoke dream-like processes in which your conscious mind doesn't have much to say. You can very well tear those pages and throw them in the garbage bin the next day...it's the energy dynamic and stress relief that matter.

The best methods to stimulate your sleep are actually meditation, relaxation exercises, and wellness programs that can put you in the right state of mind for sleep. Take a relaxing and enchanting aromatic bath with essential oils, practice massage or aromatherapy, and go for a light meditation session e.g. mindfulness meditation. Lavender, passion fruit, Melissa, mint, vanilla, sage etc. are a few plants that can help you relax and calm down your mind and your senses before going to bed.

Can exercise help you sleep better? Actually it does – provided it is practiced a few good hours before you go to bed. Jogging, running, gym, aerobics etc. ... they are all your friends when it comes to improving your sleep. They will however get you far too energized if you do these things 1-2 hours before bed time. Ideally, you should exercise in the afternoon and this it help you have an amazing energy dynamic all through the day.

You will also feel "worked up" and tired enough in the evening and your sleep will come naturally. Just keep in mind that fitness is an amazing tip for better sleep if you practice it regularly. A daily routine of around 1 hour of exercise performed 6-7 hours before you go to bed is highly recommended. As for more relaxing exercises such as yoga or stretching, you can also do them closer to your sleeping time.

Ideally you should go to bed if you're really tired. If you just force yourself to fall asleep and you lie there waiting for 1-3 hours, it might be worse and you may even get stressed out and angry. For this reason you should just engage in relaxing activities until you grow truly tired. Let your brain expend energy by engaging in light activities that will make you focus on something different from the need to fall asleep. Gradually you will get tired and actually fall asleep naturally.

Manage Your Schedule

What else can you do to make sure you sleep well? First of all, keep a healthy systematic routine and manage your daily schedule in full awareness. It's recommendable to wake up and go to bed at pretty much the same time. Maybe the exact hour will be a hard thing to respect, but you can choose your time and stick to it approximately.

For instance, you can wake up at 8-9 am every day and go to bed at 10-11 pm every night. One half an hour differences won't be harmful and it's understandable. A 4-hour shift from one day to another is prone to throwing you off balance and messing up with your sleep life. If you wake up and go to bed at close times, you will help your body and brain get accustomed to your time table and regulate its own subtle natural rhythm

To Nap or Not to Nap

Is a nap during the day an impediment to a good sleep at night? Some people might need a short nap (1-2 hours) in order to regulate their energy throughout the day. Others might notice a nap will literally 'take away' a few hours of sleep at night. If you already have your napping routine that helps you perform better at the work you have to do during the day, you can of course keep it.

However, don't forget to nap early enough so that it doesn't prevent you from falling asleep at night. 2-3 pm is a good interval for a nap. Anything after 4pm might delay your night sleep, so be careful!

Exercises for Better Sleep

For extra tips to better sleep, you can consider a few exercises that can put you in the right state of mind. Deep breathing is one of the best methods to relax before getting into bed. Dedicate 5-10 minutes to this activity every evening. Sit on your bed or lie down, close your eyes, and take deep, slow breathes while paying attention to the movement in your body.

This technique somewhat resembles mindfulness meditation, just that here the main purpose is relaxing and entering a calm mode that can you guide to slumber as opposed to activating your senses and experiencing the here and now. Another good exercise that's easy to do in bed is muscle relaxation. You should start with your toes and end with your head and face. In an initial step, you have to tighten your muscles in a specific body area.

Then let go of all the tension and let your muscles relax. To add to the efficiency of this exercise, you can play some very soft and calming music in the background e.g. classical piano music or chill out. Thus body and mind will work together towards the same goal: better sleep.

Visualizations and Affirmations

A trick that may seem amusing and unreliable at first sight is visualization. Can imagining things actually help you sleep better? Well, while the power of visualization depends a lot on one's own subconscious mind, thought control, and energetic drive, let's not ignore it! It's useful to practice visualizations for goal-reaching and promotion of positive thinking, for instance.

The law of attraction is at play during visualizations. Should you thus picture a happy person lying in bed and sleeping deeply in order to "invite" your body to sleep? Well, not really. Visualizations are more subtle than this. It's enough if you mentally picture a relaxing landscape, still water, a deep green forest etc. It's the image, the colors, and the sounds associated with what you visualize that matter. Picture yourself lying in the grass or on pillows of soft clouds. Picture yourself swaying, sailing calmly on water, or relaxing in a hammock.

Any activity that is pleasant and calming will help your mind enter the right state for sleep. If you want to add to the force of visualizations, you can also write down a number of affirmations that can make you feel at ease and unperturbed. Read them silently before you go to bed and let your mind linger on each affirmation. Meditate on their meaning and try to feel each word in your body and mind.

How to Create a Favorable

Sleeping Environment

How important is your sleeping environment for a good sleep? It's actually more important than many people think. We might tend to be superficial about it and think it's enough to lie down on a horizontal surface that's comfortable enough … and sleep will just come to you. In fact, you have to "invite" your sleep by means of environment optimization. How can you do this?

Preparing the Perfect Bed

First of all, you should only sleep on a smooth mattress, soft pillows, nice-smelling sheets, smooth blankets etc. Any detail that's harsh to the touch and unpleasant to any other sense will hinder your sleep, although you may not even realize it consciously.

You might not realize you don't actually like the far too chemical smell of your pillow cases or the starchy feel of your sheets. Such details can easily go unnoticed, especially if for some people they appear "normal". But it's enough that your body or brain dislikes something … and this minor detail can affect your sleep.

The ideal colors for your beddings are soft and sweet pink, light blue, lavender, green, light yellow, grey, or cream. Some people might be fans of intricate patterns and color combinations. While that can be quite fascinating as design, it may not actually be very beneficial to your sleep and mood. Choose a more simple kind of bedding with tranquil colors and feel. Avoid totally white linen, as it is too much evocative of a hospital-like atmosphere.

Go for something silky and fine to the touch. If you want to add more "spice" to your sleeping environment, feel free to use a roll to put behind your neck, a wedge to place behind your back, one or two more elegant small pillows only to make your space more lively and inviting, and even a teddy bear or another "communicative" figure that can make you feel more intimate and at rest in your own bed.

Keeping Your Room Tidy

Make sure your room looks good and is very tidy. Dust, disorder, unpleasant smells, or just the presence of microbes one way or another in your room are likely to make your sleep less pleasant and easy. Again ...you might not notice it right away, but your sleep can be influenced in a rather indirect way. That's why you should always keep your room clean and full of fresh air. It's actually quite essential to allow a lot of fresh air in your room right before you go to bed. If the air outside is not too cold, you will just benefit from a well oxygenated room.

The Energy of Your Room

Make sure you manage the energy in your room well enough. It's advisable to keep your work materials out of your sleeping environment. Of course, some people may have to use the same room for both sleep and work. In this case, you should at least place your bed in a comfortable corner and don't mix that area up with your work 'apparel'. Ideally your computer, your professional books and files, and your work attire should be far away.

In most cases, people can afford having a full bedroom at hand just to rest and sleep in. In this case, maybe it's better to also keep your TV set out of the room you save for sleep. You can watch TV in your living room. Pay attention to many details in your bedroom – from wall color and furniture to smell/perfume. Don't fill your bedroom with too much furniture – it should look spacey and inviting, not like an old forgotten attic where things are stuck and piled for ages.

Why does the paint on your walls matter? You actually keep your eyes closed when you want to sleep , you don't stare at the walls, don't you? This is true. However, the colors in your bedroom matter because of the vibe and atmosphere they create. People instinctively associate a space with a specific mood or energy, even if they might not literally think or talk about it.

The energy of an environment does enter their subconscious mind and it makes them feel one way or another. A very dark room with a Gothic air might not be the best idea for a sleeping environment. Similarly, a very stridently colored room whose walls are magenta or fuchsia might cause some mental strain that's not propitious for sleep. It's not your actual mood when you lie down in your bed to sleep we're talking about here! It's the energy inherent in a room that can be favorable to rest and replenishing sleep or can subvert your need to relax have a good sleep. Which are the ideal colors for a good sleep?

Light blue and green are probably the best idea. These colors are calming and soothing to the human mind and they add a refreshing hue to any space. Light pink and yellow, white to cream, and peach are also recommendable colors for your bedroom. They will fill your sleeping environment with both positive and chill energy.

The Right Light/Darkness Balance

A very significant aspect is light. Your sleeping environment should follow the natural light flow. You should expose yourself to enough sunlight during the day and adapt slowly to a softer kind of light that respects natural changes, even though it's artificial. Ideally, you should keep your circadian rhythm in check by spending time in corresponding environments.

Make sure you have enough natural bright light in your room as and after you wake up and spend enough time enjoying sunlight. Towards the evening, you should avoid strong, intense light in the evening. Simply purchase the right kind of light bulb. Something bright might be good when you have to spend time at your desk and work. However, use only soft, calming light in your bedroom. If you read before you go to bed, don't use light that's too intense. It's better to use a lamp that's closer to your bed and provides you with warm, soft light rather than only rely of the more intense light spreading from your ceiling.

You can perfectly regulate your exposure to light by spending enough time during the day in sunlight and avoiding any source of bright light before sleep time. How can you do this? It's not only light sources that matter. You should also avoid bright screens within 2 hours of going to bed. That's why it's not advisable to watch TV or work on your computer too late or at least not right before you want to go to bed.

The artificial light will affect you without knowing. If you really have to use your laptop or your tablet, you can at least adjust the light and brightness to suit that specific moment of the day. When you actually have to fall asleep, make sure your room is as dark as possible after you turn off the lights. Use heavy curtains and shades to block any light during the night. Avoid keeping in your room electronic devices that emit light e.g. digital clock, charging phone etc. They can disturb you in an insidious way. If it's inevitable to wake up at night (e.g. in order to drink some water out of obvious thirst or in order go to the restroom), try to keep the lights off as much as possible. Any abrupt and intense light will affect your natural rhythm and your sleep afterwards.

Noise

Similarly, anything that produces noise should be removed from your sleeping environment. Make sure you have no fridge or loud clock around you to mess with your sleep. Keep your windows tightly closed and make sure you don't have a bed that produces some noise when you turn or toss in your bed unwillingly. It will bother you even when it won't wake you up fully.

Temperature

Temperature is also an important factor in your sleeping environment. Keep your room cool enough and let fresh air in as often as possible. Does a warm room mess with your sleep? While a warm room is very comfortable for some and is actually recommended for your health to avoid cold and damp environments, keep in mind the most suitable temperature for a great sleeping environment is around 18 degrees. Good ventilation is also recommendable if you want to sleep well.

That said a room that's slightly cool will provide you with the perfect sleeping atmosphere as long as you get dressed adequately and cover yourself with a warm blanket. You shouldn't feel cold at night. However, your environment should be cool enough. Some studies have shown that keeping your limbs warm will help you fall asleep easier. For this purpose you can use some thick, warm socks that you put on when you get into bed. Keep your hands warm by means of massage or warm water.

Keep Your Bed Only For Its Natural Purposes

Your bed should be kept only for sleep … and sex. You should allow for no other activity to be associated with your actual sleeping space. Avoid working in bed or reading 'heavy' material for work. Don't eat on your bed and don't use it as a sitting place for people you have conversation with in your home. Simply save your bed for its primary purpose: sleep. Thus your mind will almost automatically get into 'sleeping mode' as you approach this area of your house. It won't ring 'hard task' or 'stressful energy' by any means and all your memories will center on sleeping-related activities.

No Pets in Your Bed

If you have pets, the best advice is to keep them out of your bed. Of course during daytime they might jump and mingle with you as you move around the house. However, it's for your own benefit to keep your cat or your dog away from your sleeping environment, as they will only add an element of unpredictability and maybe even noise that you don't really need. Train your pets to stay out of your bed. This will also ensure you don't provoke allergies and disturb your sleep even more.

Use Separate Sheets

If you sleep with your partner (or a sister/child), it's recommendable to use separate sheets and blankets so as not to 'fight' over warmth and comfort during the night. Maybe that will decrease the feeling of intimacy if you sleep with your partner, but it's more likely to ensure you have a good and pleasant sleeping environment only for yourself. Your mind or heart might need to be very close to your partner physically, but your body also needs to have an oasis of its own and not share too much space with another. This way you don't risk running out of blanket and getting too cold during the night. The sensation of sudden coldness will most likely wake you up.

Pillows

Your pillow is quite important to good sleep. What kind of pillow do you need? If you are allergic to feathers or wool, you have to avoid such items at any cost. Don't even keep them in your room, as they will make you sneeze or cough at night. It doesn't matter that your partner is not allergic. Keep any harmful element completely out of your room. What size is optimal? Ideally your pillow should be soft, but full enough. You need to rest your head on an even, cozy surface and not just have something pushed under your head. Use a moderately large pillow that doesn't make you hold your head too high and your neck too bent.

The best pillow is not very tick, but medium-sized and consistent. Some people have learned to do without a pillow. That's not a rule for all, but you should know it's actually something good for one's neck and back. However, if you notice you cannot sleep well without a pillow, don't sacrifice your rest only to have fewer neck wrinkles or perfect upper back health. There's no one-size-fits all when it comes to what one finds comfortable to sleep on. In any case, huge and heavy pillows that cover too much space and make you twist your neck should be avoided.

Your Sleeping Position

What about your sleeping position? Is there any that are harmful or subversive of your sleep? The idea sleeping postures imply a rather straight body and keeping one's limbs free from weight or strain. That's why many specialists recommend sleeping on your back on your side. Stomach sleepers might have a harder time on the long run, as their face wrinkles more easily and their hands might get numb during the night. Sleeping on one's back seems to be the best tip for your overall health and comfort.

But we all know sometimes it gets hard to stick to one position only, as the body needs change and avoidance of muscle strain. Switch to sleeping on the side, but don't keep your arm bent under your ear, as you might damage your nerves. Try to keep your neck and your back straight as much as possible.
Some people noticed that putting one's feet up on a higher surface located on the bed or right next to the bed is better for

sleep. From a strictly medical point of view, this explains through a form of 'cleansing' of your legs of the blood and lymph that gather there during the day and can affect cortisol levels. Psychologically this position is also good, because it simply reverts your daily body posture.

You may be lying in bed horizontally at night …but keeping your legs in an angle in relation to your body will simply invoke another state in your brain. Alternatively, you can only practice this position as a relaxing technique before falling asleep. You can use your bed and place your legs on many pillows or you can lie on the floor and raise your legs on your bed. The point is having a 90 degree angle in this posture. You can let your legs rest like this for 30 minutes or more while you read a book, listen to some music, or enjoy an audio program that can help you relax and feel good.

Clothing

What kind of clothes should you use in bed? Is there a rule to follow? Sleeping naked is said to be quite good for our bodies and sleep, but many people might find it weird and hard to get used to. You should try it and test your body comfort. Use smooth and silky bedding and sheets and let your skin sink in the magnetizing feeling.

Make sure your blankets are thick enough to keep you warm. If you don't tolerate sleeping naked too well, the classic pajamas or nightgown are also good enough as long as the fabric is high quality and it doesn't make you sweat or leave you too cold during the night. Adjust your clothes to your room temperature. It's better to use lighter clothes and a blanket that's warm enough, as your body will be able to breathe more freely this way.

A Sanctuary for the Senses

To enhance the pleasantness of your sleeping sanctuary, you can also use scent that appeals to the senses and work on your mind at the same time. Lavender, vanilla, rosemary, opium, rose, orange blossom, jasmine, or coconut oil are just a few suggestions. Use essential oils and prepare a spray that you can enliven your sleeping environment with.

The herbal essences will act on your mind and help you relax and your space will smell wonderfully. Loving your sleeping sanctuary is a vital part of getting a good sleep. Don't just treat your bedroom as a 'necessary evil', the place where you 'have to' go to sleep in. Do your best to turn your sleep into a real ritual and mind all the small or significant details that can enhance the coziness, hygiene, freshness, and pleasantness of your environment.

You can also light scented candles or place raw essential oil in a recipient on your desk or your night commode. The scent will help you rest well and fall asleep in an enchanting atmosphere.

Conclusions

This book introduced you to what good sleep means, why you should care about healthy sleeping habits, and how you can improve your sleep. As already suggested, if you find yourself suffering from severe insomnia that strikes you regularly regardless of what you do during the day, it's recommendable to consult a medical specialist before resorting to the tips in this book.

 Sleeping disorders might have a deeper cause and be one side of an underlying health condition such as anemia, depression, hormone imbalances, thyroid dysfunction, nervous disturbances, anxiety/panic disorders etc. If your sleeping problems are persistent, it's vital that you investigate all the problems and connect the dots before you start treating your sleep. After you get professional advice and even treatment through medication, you are always welcome to practice all the tips in this book.

If you only have sleeping difficulties once in a while, you find it hard to fall asleep, you wake up without any reason during the night, or you feel you don't get enough rest in general, this short guide to better sleep is your right ally! Keep in mind that you have to practice all the techniques and tips presented in this book within a more general program based on a holistic approach. It's not enough to pay attention to your sleeping environment if you totally ignore diet aspects, for instance.

Try to integrate all the advice in this book into your daily routines and you will see that your sleep improves considerably!

www.ingramcontent.com/pod-product-compliance
Lightning Source LLC
Chambersburg PA
CBHW071306280526
45788CB00004B/1843